CKD STAGE 4 COOKBOOK FOR VEGANS

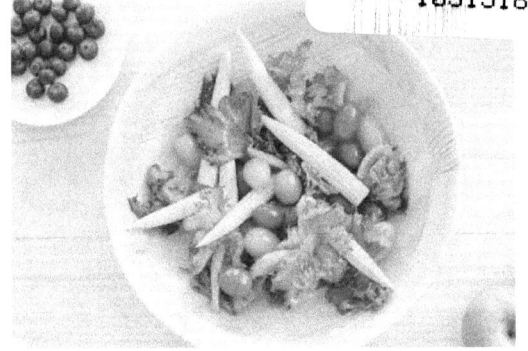

DR. JESSICA SMITH

Copyright © 2024 by DR. JESSICA SMITH

All rights reserved.

No part of this book may be reproduced, stored in a retrieval system, or transmitted, in any form or by any means, electronic, mechanical, photocopying, recording, or otherwise, without prior written permission from the publisher, except for brief quotations embodied in critical articles or reviews.

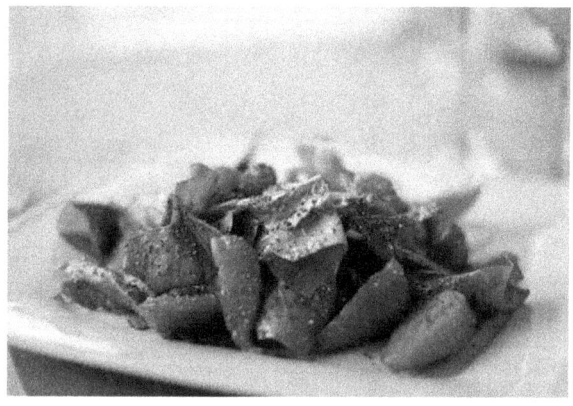

TABLE OF CONTENTS

CHAPTER ONE 7

How to Use this Cookbook 7

Understanding Ckd Stage 4 Cookbook for Vegans .. 9

Benefits of Ckd Stage 4 Cookbook for Vegans 10

Guidelines for Ckd Stage 4 Cookbook for Vegans. 12

CHAPTER TWO 15

CKD Stage 4 Breakfast Recipes for Vegans 15

1: Quinoa Breakfast Bowl 15

2: Avocado Toast with Spinach and Tomato 16

3: Oatmeal with Mixed Berries and Almond Butter 18

4: Tofu Scramble with Vegetables 20

5: Chia Seed Pudding with Mango and Coconut ... 22

6: Sweet Potato Breakfast Hash 23

7: Berry Smoothie Bowl 25

8: Buckwheat Pancakes with Mixed Fruit Compote 27

9: Spinach and Mushroom Tofu Scramble 30

10: Vegan Breakfast Burrito 32

CKD Stage 4 Lunch Recipes for Vegans 34

1: Lentil and Vegetable Soup 34

2: Chickpea Salad Wraps 36

3: Quinoa Salad with Roasted Vegetables 38

5: Stuffed Bell Peppers with Quinoa and Black Beans 44

6: Mediterranean Chickpea Salad 46

7: Vegan Lentil Salad 48

8: Vegan Mediterranean Wrap 50

9: Vegan Mediterranean Pasta Salad 52

10: Vegan Bean and Vegetable Soup 54

CKD Stage 4 Dinner Recipes for Vegans 57

1: Vegan Chickpea Curry 57

2: Vegan Lentil Shepherd's Pie 59

3: Vegan Quinoa Stuffed Bell Peppers 62

4: Vegan Lentil and Vegetable Stir-Fry 65

5: Vegan Eggplant and Lentil Moussaka 68

6: Vegan Mediterranean Stuffed Acorn Squash 71

7: Vegan Lentil Shepherd's Pie 74

8: Vegan Mediterranean Stuffed Portobello Mushrooms 77

9: Vegan Lentil and Vegetable Soup 79

10: Vegan Quinoa and Vegetable Stir-Fry 81

CKD Stage 4 Snacks Recipes for Vegans 83

1: Vegan Hummus and Vegetable Platter 83

2: Vegan Avocado Toast 85

3: Vegan Berry Smoothie Bowl 87

4: Vegan Antipasto Skewers 89

5: Vegan Chickpea Salad 90

6: Vegan Rice Cake with Almond Butter and Banana 92
7: Vegan Stuffed Mini Bell Peppers 94
8: Vegan Greek Yogurt Parfait 96
9: Vegan Edamame Salad 97
10: Vegan Chia Pudding 99
CONCLUSION 102

CHAPTER ONE

How to Use this Cookbook

Understand Your Dietary Restrictions: Before diving into the cookbook, familiarize yourself with your dietary restrictions as per your CKD Stage 4 condition. This will help you make informed choices while selecting recipes.

Gather Necessary Ingredients: Take stock of the ingredients you have and make a shopping list for the ones you need. Ensure they align with your dietary requirements and restrictions.

Browse Recipes: Take your time to flip through this cookbook and mark recipes that catch your eye. Look for dishes that incorporate kidney-friendly ingredients and align with your taste preferences.

Check Nutritional Information: Pay attention to the nutritional information provided for each recipe. Look for recipes that are low in sodium, phosphorus, and potassium, as these are often restricted in CKD diets.

Plan Your Meals: Once you've selected recipes, plan your meals for the week accordingly. Consider factors like variety, balance, and portion sizes to ensure you're meeting your nutritional needs.

Prepare Meals Mindfully: When cooking, follow the recipes closely and be mindful of portion sizes and ingredient substitutions if necessary.

Opt for cooking methods that are kidney-friendly, such as boiling, steaming, or baking.

Monitor Your Intake: Keep track of your food and fluid intake to ensure you're adhering to your dietary restrictions. Consider using a food journal or app to help you stay organized.

Listen to Your Body: Pay attention to how your body responds to different foods and adjust your diet as needed. If you experience any adverse effects or symptoms, consult with your healthcare provider.

Stay Informed: Continuously educate yourself about CKD Stage 4 and vegan nutrition to make informed decisions about your diet.

Stay updated on new recipes, cooking techniques, and dietary guidelines to support your kidney health.

Understanding Ckd Stage 4 Cookbook for Vegans

Understanding a CKD Stage 4 Cookbook tailored for vegans requires insight into both chronic kidney disease (CKD) management and vegan nutrition.

CKD Stage 4 signifies a severe reduction in kidney function, necessitating careful dietary choices to manage symptoms and slow disease progression.

Meanwhile, a vegan diet excludes all animal products, emphasizing plant-based foods rich in nutrients and fiber.

This specialized cookbook integrates both aspects, offering recipes designed to support kidney health while adhering to vegan principles.

It typically emphasizes foods low in sodium, phosphorus, and potassium, as these are often restricted in CKD diets to prevent complications like high blood pressure and electrolyte imbalances. Furthermore, it highlights plant-based sources of protein, such as legumes, tofu, and quinoa, which are essential for muscle repair and overall health in CKD patients.

This cookbook may also provide guidance on portion sizes, meal planning, and ingredient substitutions to accommodate individual dietary needs and preferences. Understanding the nuances of CKD Stage 4 and vegan nutrition empowers individuals to make informed choices when selecting recipes and preparing meals.

By following the cookbook's recommendations and consulting with healthcare professionals as needed, individuals can effectively manage their condition while enjoying delicious, kidney-friendly vegan dishes.

Benefits of Ckd Stage 4 Cookbook for Vegans

A CKD Stage 4 Cookbook tailored for vegans offers several distinct benefits for individuals managing chronic kidney disease (CKD) in its advanced stages while adhering to a vegan lifestyle.

Firstly, such a cookbook provides a comprehensive resource specifically tailored to the dietary needs and restrictions of individuals with CKD Stage 4 who choose to follow a vegan diet. It offers a variety of recipes that are not only delicious but also carefully crafted to support kidney health by focusing on ingredients low in sodium, phosphorus, and potassium, which are typically restricted in CKD diets to prevent complications such as fluid retention and electrolyte imbalances.

Moreover, a CKD Stage 4 Cookbook for Vegans promotes the consumption of nutrient-dense plant-based foods that are rich in antioxidants, vitamins, and minerals, which can help mitigate inflammation, oxidative stress, and other factors contributing to kidney damage. By emphasizing whole grains, fruits, vegetables, and plant-based sources of protein, the cookbook encourages a balanced and diverse diet that supports overall health and well-being.

The cookbook facilitates meal planning and preparation, making it easier for individuals with CKD Stage 4 to adhere to their dietary regimen while enjoying flavorful and satisfying meals.

It also fosters creativity in the kitchen, empowering individuals to explore new ingredients and cooking techniques that align with both their dietary needs and personal taste preferences.

A CKD Stage 4 Cookbook for Vegans serves as a valuable tool for individuals seeking to optimize their nutritional intake, manage their condition effectively, and enhance their quality of life through delicious and kidney-friendly plant-based meals.

Guidelines for Ckd Stage 4 Cookbook for Vegans

Guidelines for utilizing a CKD Stage 4 Cookbook for Vegans provide essential direction for individuals managing advanced chronic kidney disease (CKD) while following a vegan diet.

These guidelines serve as a roadmap for making informed dietary choices and optimizing kidney health through plant-based nutrition.

Understand Dietary Restrictions: Familiarize yourself with the dietary restrictions associated with CKD Stage 4, including limitations on sodium, phosphorus, and potassium intake. Ensure recipes in the cookbook aligns with these restrictions.

Focus on Nutrient-Rich Foods: Emphasize nutrient-dense plant-based foods, such as fruits, vegetables, whole grains, legumes, and nuts, which provide essential vitamins, minerals, and antioxidants to support kidney function and overall health.

Limit High-Potassium Ingredients: Be mindful of ingredients high in potassium, such as bananas, potatoes, and tomatoes. Opt for lower potassium alternatives or moderate portion sizes to avoid exceeding daily intake limits.

Choose Low-Phosphorus Options: Select recipes featuring ingredients low in phosphorus to prevent complications associated with elevated phosphorus levels, such as bone and cardiovascular issues. Examples include rice, pasta, and non-dairy milk alternatives.

Reduce Sodium Content: Minimize the use of added salt and choose low-sodium or salt-free seasonings and condiments to control blood pressure and fluid retention.

Flavor dishes with herbs, spices, citrus juice, and vinegar instead.

Balance Protein Intake: Incorporate plant-based sources of protein, such as beans, lentils, tofu, tempeh, and seitan, into your meals to support muscle health and repair without overloading the kidneys with excess protein.

Monitor Fluid Intake: Keep track of fluid intake as per your healthcare provider's recommendations to prevent fluid overload and maintain electrolyte balance.

Choose hydrating foods like cucumbers, lettuce, and watermelon while limiting high-fluid foods like soups and stews.

Seek Professional Guidance: Consult with a registered dietitian or healthcare provider specializing in kidney health to tailor the cookbook's recommendations to your individual dietary needs and medical condition.

Experiment with Recipes: Explore the cookbook's diverse range of recipes and adapt them to suit your taste preferences and dietary requirements. Don't hesitate to experiment with ingredient substitutions and cooking methods to enhance flavor and nutritional value.

Practice Portion Control: Pay attention to portion sizes to avoid overeating and ensure balanced nutrient intake. Use measuring cups, spoons, and food scales as needed to maintain portion control and monitor caloric and nutrient intake.

CHAPTER TWO

CKD Stage 4 Breakfast Recipes for Vegans

1: Quinoa Breakfast Bowl

Ingredients:

- 1/2 cup quinoa
- 1 cup almond milk (unsweetened)
- 1 tablespoon chia seeds
- 1/2 cup mixed berries (blueberries, strawberries, raspberries)
- 1 tablespoon chopped nuts (almonds, walnuts)
- 1 teaspoon maple syrup (optional)

Detailed Instructions:

- Rinse the quinoa under cold water.
- In a small saucepan, combine the quinoa and almond milk. Bring to a boil, then reduce heat to low, cover, and simmer for 15 minutes or until quinoa is cooked and fluffy.
- Stir in the chia seeds and let it sit for 5 minutes to thicken.

- Divide the cooked quinoa into bowls.
- Top each bowl with mixed berries and chopped nuts.
- Drizzle with maple syrup if desired.
- Serve warm and enjoy!

Health Benefits:

- Quinoa is a complete protein, providing all nine essential amino acids, which is beneficial for muscle health.
- Berries are rich in antioxidants, vitamins, and fiber, supporting overall health and reducing inflammation.
- Chia seeds are high in omega-3 fatty acids and fiber, promoting heart health and aiding digestion.
- Almond milk is low in potassium and phosphorus, making it a kidney-friendly alternative to dairy milk.

Preparation Time: Approximately 20 minutes.

2: Avocado Toast with Spinach and Tomato

Ingredients:

- 2 slices whole grain bread (low-sodium)
- 1 ripe avocado

- 1 cup fresh spinach leaves
- 1 medium tomato, sliced
- 1 teaspoon lemon juice
- Salt and pepper to taste

Detailed Instructions:

- Toast the whole grain bread slices until golden brown.
- Mash the ripe avocado in a bowl and mix with lemon juice, salt, and pepper.
- Spread the mashed avocado evenly onto each toast slice.
- Top each toast with fresh spinach leaves and tomato slices.
- Season with additional salt and pepper if desired.
- Serve immediately.

Health Benefits:

- Whole grain bread is high in fiber and complex carbohydrates, providing sustained energy and promoting digestive health.

- Avocado is rich in healthy fats, vitamins, and minerals, supporting heart health and reducing inflammation.
- Spinach is low in potassium and phosphorus, making it an excellent choice for kidney health.
- Tomatoes are a good source of antioxidants, vitamins, and lycopene, which may help protect against certain chronic diseases.

Preparation Time: Approximately 10 minutes.

3: Oatmeal with Mixed Berries and Almond Butter

Ingredients:

- 1/2 cup rolled oats (steel-cut or quick oats)
- 1 cup water
- 1/2 cup mixed berries (blueberries, strawberries, raspberries)
- 1 tablespoon almond butter
- 1 teaspoon maple syrup (optional)
- Pinch of cinnamon (optional)

Detailed Instructions:

- In a small saucepan, bring water to a boil.
- Stir in the rolled oats and reduce heat to low.
- Cook the oats, stirring occasionally, for 5-7 minutes or until thickened to your desired consistency.
- Once cooked, transfer the oatmeal to a bowl.
- Top with mixed berries and a dollop of almond butter.
- Drizzle with maple syrup and sprinkle with cinnamon if desired.
- Serve warm and enjoy!

Health Benefits:

- Oats are rich in soluble fiber, which helps lower cholesterol levels and stabilize blood sugar levels.
- Mixed berries are packed with antioxidants and vitamins, supporting immune function and reducing inflammation.
- Almond butter provides healthy fats, protein, and fiber, promoting satiety and heart health.

- Maple syrup adds sweetness without refined sugars and is lower in potassium compared to other sweeteners.

Preparation Time: Approximately 10 minutes.

4: Tofu Scramble with Vegetables

Ingredients:

- 200g firm tofu, crumbled
- 1/2 cup diced bell peppers (red, green, yellow)
- 1/4 cup diced onion
- 1/2 cup chopped spinach
- 1 clove garlic, minced
- 1 tablespoon nutritional yeast
- 1/2 teaspoon turmeric powder
- Salt and pepper to taste
- 1 teaspoon olive oil

Detailed Instructions:

- Heat olive oil in a skillet over medium heat.
- Add minced garlic and diced onion, sauté until softened.

- Add diced bell peppers and chopped spinach, cook until vegetables are tender.
- Crumble the tofu into the skillet and sprinkle with turmeric powder and nutritional yeast.
- Cook, stirring occasionally, for 5-7 minutes or until tofu is heated through and lightly browned.
- Season with salt and pepper to taste.
- Serve hot with whole grain toast or tortillas.

Health Benefits:

- Tofu is a plant-based source of protein, low in potassium and phosphorus, and supports muscle health and repair.
- Bell peppers are rich in vitamin C and antioxidants, promoting immune function and reducing inflammation.
- Spinach provides iron and folate, essential for red blood cell production and overall health.
- Nutritional yeast adds a cheesy flavor and is a source of B vitamins, particularly important for vegans.

Preparation Time: Approximately 15 minutes.

5: Chia Seed Pudding with Mango and Coconut

Ingredients:

- 2 tablespoons chia seeds
- 1/2 cup unsweetened coconut milk
- 1/2 teaspoon vanilla extract
- 1/2 ripe mango, diced
- 1 tablespoon shredded coconut (unsweetened)
- 1 teaspoon agave syrup or maple syrup (optional)

Detailed Instructions:

- In a bowl, combine chia seeds, coconut milk, and vanilla extract. Stir well to combine.
- Cover the bowl and refrigerate for at least 2 hours or overnight, allowing the chia seeds to absorb the liquid and form a pudding-like consistency.
- Once the chia pudding is set, remove it from the refrigerator and give it a stir.
- Divide the pudding into serving glasses or bowls.
- Top each serving with diced mango and shredded coconut.
- Drizzle with agave syrup or maple syrup if desired.
- Serve chilled and enjoy!

Health Benefits:

- Chia seeds are rich in fiber, omega-3 fatty acids, and protein, supporting digestive health and heart health.
- Coconut milk adds creaminess and provides medium-chain triglycerides (MCTs), which may have potential benefits for brain health and weight management.
- Mangoes are high in vitamin C, vitamin A, and antioxidants, supporting immune function and skin health.
- Shredded coconut adds flavor and texture without adding significant amounts of potassium or phosphorus.

Preparation Time: Approximately 5 minutes (plus chilling time).

6: Sweet Potato Breakfast Hash

Ingredients:

- 1 medium sweet potato, peeled and diced
- 1/2 cup diced bell peppers (any color)
- 1/4 cup diced onion

- 1/2 cup cooked black beans (canned, rinsed and drained)
- 1 teaspoon olive oil
- 1/2 teaspoon smoked paprika
- Salt and pepper to taste
- Fresh cilantro or parsley for garnish (optional)

Detailed Instructions:

- Heat olive oil in a skillet over medium heat.
- Add diced sweet potato and cook for 5-7 minutes, stirring occasionally, until slightly softened.
- Add diced bell peppers and onion to the skillet, continue cooking until vegetables are tender.
- Stir in cooked black beans and smoked paprika, cooking for an additional 2-3 minutes to heat through.
- Season with salt and pepper to taste.
- Remove from heat and garnish with fresh cilantro or parsley if desired.
- Serve hot as is or with a side of whole grain toast.

Health Benefits:

- Sweet potatoes are rich in vitamins A and C, fiber, and antioxidants, supporting eye health and immune function.
- Black beans are a good source of plant-based protein, fiber, and folate, promoting digestive health and cardiovascular health.
- Bell peppers add color and flavor while providing vitamin C and antioxidants, supporting skin health and immune function.
- Olive oil provides healthy fats and adds richness to the dish without significantly increasing sodium or phosphorus content.

Preparation Time: Approximately 20 minutes.

7: Berry Smoothie Bowl

Ingredients:

- 1 cup mixed berries (strawberries, blueberries, raspberries)
- 1 ripe banana, sliced
- 1/2 cup unsweetened almond milk

- 1 tablespoon chia seeds
- 1 tablespoon hemp seeds
- 1 tablespoon almond butter
- Toppings: sliced fresh fruit, shredded coconut, granola (optional)

Detailed Instructions:

- In a blender, combine mixed berries, banana slices, almond milk, chia seeds, hemp seeds, and almond butter.
- Blend until smooth and creamy, adding more almond milk if needed to reach desired consistency.
- Pour the smoothie into a bowl.
- Top with sliced fresh fruit, shredded coconut, and granola if desired.
- Serve immediately with a spoon and enjoy!

Health Benefits:

- Berries are rich in antioxidants, fiber, and vitamins, supporting heart health and reducing inflammation.

- Bananas provide potassium and vitamin B6, which help regulate blood pressure and support nerve function.
- Chia seeds and hemp seeds are excellent sources of omega-3 fatty acids, protein, and fiber, promoting satiety and digestive health.
- Almond butter adds creaminess and healthy fats without increasing sodium or phosphorus levels significantly.

Preparation Time: Approximately 5 minutes.

8: Buckwheat Pancakes with Mixed Fruit Compote

Ingredients:

For the pancakes:

- 1 cup buckwheat flour
- 1 tablespoon ground flaxseed
- 1 teaspoon baking powder
- 1/2 teaspoon cinnamon
- 1 cup unsweetened almond milk
- 1 tablespoon maple syrup (optional)

- 1 teaspoon vanilla extract
- Cooking spray or coconut oil for greasing

For the fruit compote:

- 1 cup mixed fruit (such as berries, peaches, or apples), diced
- 1 tablespoon lemon juice
- 1 tablespoon maple syrup (optional)
- 1/2 teaspoon vanilla extract

Detailed Instructions:

- In a mixing bowl, whisk together buckwheat flour, ground flaxseed, baking powder, and cinnamon.
- In a separate bowl, mix almond milk, maple syrup (if using), and vanilla extract.
- Gradually pour the wet ingredients into the dry ingredients, stirring until just combined. Do not overmix.
- Heat a non-stick skillet or griddle over medium heat and lightly grease with cooking spray or coconut oil.

- Pour about 1/4 cup of batter onto the skillet for each pancake. Cook until bubbles form on the surface, then flip and cook until golden brown on both sides.
- Meanwhile, prepare the fruit compote by combining mixed fruit, lemon juice, maple syrup (if using), and vanilla extract in a saucepan. Cook over medium heat for 5-7 minutes, or until the fruit is softened and the mixture has thickened slightly.
- Serve the buckwheat pancakes topped with the mixed fruit compote.
- Optionally, garnish with a dollop of coconut yogurt or a sprinkle of chopped nuts.

Health Benefits:

- Buckwheat flour is gluten-free and rich in fiber, protein, and minerals such as manganese and magnesium, supporting digestive health and blood sugar control.
- Ground flaxseed adds omega-3 fatty acids and lignans, which have anti-inflammatory and antioxidant properties.

- Mixed fruits provide vitamins, minerals, and antioxidants, contributing to overall health and immune function.
- Maple syrup adds natural sweetness without refined sugars and is lower in potassium compared to other sweeteners.

Preparation Time: Approximately 30 minutes.

9: Spinach and Mushroom Tofu Scramble

Ingredients:

- 200g firm tofu, crumbled
- 1 cup fresh spinach leaves, chopped
- 1/2 cup sliced mushrooms
- 1/4 cup diced onion
- 1 clove garlic, minced
- 1 tablespoon nutritional yeast
- 1/2 teaspoon turmeric powder
- Salt and pepper to taste
- 1 teaspoon olive oil

Detailed Instructions:

- Heat olive oil in a skillet over medium heat.
- Add minced garlic and diced onion, sauté until softened.
- Add sliced mushrooms and chopped spinach to the skillet, cook until vegetables are tender.
- Crumble the tofu into the skillet and sprinkle with turmeric powder and nutritional yeast.
- Cook, stirring occasionally, for 5-7 minutes or until tofu is heated through and lightly browned.
- Season with salt and pepper to taste.
- Serve hot with whole grain toast or tortillas.

Health Benefits:

- Tofu is a plant-based source of protein, low in potassium and phosphorus, and supports muscle health and repair.
- Spinach is low in potassium and phosphorus and provides iron and vitamin K, which are essential for blood and bone health.

- Mushrooms are low in potassium and provide antioxidants and B vitamins, supporting immune function and energy metabolism.
- Nutritional yeast adds a cheesy flavor and is a source of B vitamins, particularly important for vegans.

Preparation Time: Approximately 15 minutes.

10: Vegan Breakfast Burrito

Ingredients:

- 1/2 cup cooked quinoa
- 1/2 cup black beans, cooked or canned (rinsed and drained)
- 1/4 cup diced bell peppers (any color)
- 1/4 cup diced onion
- 1/2 avocado, sliced
- 2 whole grain tortillas
- 1 tablespoon salsa (optional)
- Fresh cilantro for garnish (optional)
- Lime wedges for serving

Detailed Instructions:

- In a skillet, heat cooked quinoa, black beans, diced bell peppers, and diced onion until warmed through.
- Warm the tortillas in the skillet or microwave for a few seconds to make them pliable.
- Divide the quinoa and black bean mixture between the tortillas.
- Top each tortilla with sliced avocado and salsa if desired.
- Garnish with fresh cilantro.
- Roll up the tortillas into burritos.
- Serve with lime wedges for squeezing over the burritos.

Health Benefits:

- Quinoa is a complete protein and a good source of fiber, supporting muscle health and digestive health.
- Black beans are rich in protein, fiber, and folate, promoting satiety and cardiovascular health.
- Bell peppers provide vitamin C and antioxidants, supporting immune function and reducing inflammation.

- Avocado adds healthy fats and potassium, which may help lower blood pressure and reduce the risk of heart disease.

Preparation Time: Approximately 20 minutes.

CKD Stage 4 Lunch Recipes for Vegans

1: Lentil and Vegetable Soup

Ingredients:

- 1 cup dried green or brown lentils, rinsed
- 4 cups low-sodium vegetable broth
- 1 cup diced carrots
- 1 cup diced celery
- 1 cup diced onion
- 2 cloves garlic, minced
- 1 teaspoon dried thyme
- 1 teaspoon dried rosemary
- Salt and pepper to taste
- 2 tablespoons chopped fresh parsley for garnish (optional)

Detailed Instructions:

- In a large pot, combine the lentils, vegetable broth, diced carrots, diced celery, diced onion, minced garlic, dried thyme, and dried rosemary.
- Bring the mixture to a boil over medium-high heat, then reduce the heat to low, cover, and simmer for 20-25 minutes or until the lentils and vegetables are tender.
- Season the soup with salt and pepper to taste.
- Ladle the soup into bowls and garnish with chopped fresh parsley if desired.
- Serve hot with whole grain bread or crackers.

Health Benefits:

- Lentils are a good source of plant-based protein, fiber, and iron, supporting muscle health, digestive health, and energy levels.
- Carrots, celery, and onions are rich in vitamins, minerals, and antioxidants, promoting immune function and reducing inflammation.

- Garlic contains compounds with antibacterial and anti-inflammatory properties, supporting heart health and immune function.
- Fresh parsley adds flavor and is a good source of vitamin K and antioxidants, supporting bone health and reducing oxidative stress.

Preparation Time: Approximately 30 minutes.

2: Chickpea Salad Wraps

Ingredients:

For the chickpea salad:

- 1 can (15 ounces) chickpeas, rinsed and drained
- 1/4 cup diced red bell pepper
- 1/4 cup diced cucumber
- 2 tablespoons diced red onion
- 2 tablespoons chopped fresh parsley
- 2 tablespoons lemon juice
- 1 tablespoon olive oil
- Salt and pepper to taste

For assembling wraps:

- 4 large whole grain tortillas
- 1 cup baby spinach leaves
- 1/2 avocado, sliced
- 1/4 cup hummus (optional)

Detailed Instructions:

- In a mixing bowl, mash the chickpeas with a fork or potato masher until slightly chunky.
- Add diced red bell pepper, diced cucumber, diced red onion, chopped fresh parsley, lemon juice, olive oil, salt, and pepper to the mashed chickpeas. Mix well to combine.
- Lay out the whole grain tortillas on a flat surface.
- Spread a layer of baby spinach leaves on each tortilla.
- Spoon the chickpea salad mixture onto the spinach leaves.
- Top each wrap with sliced avocado and a dollop of hummus if desired.
- Roll up the wraps tightly, folding in the sides as you go.
- Slice the wraps in half diagonally and serve.

Health Benefits:

- Chickpeas are a good source of protein, fiber, and folate, supporting muscle health, digestive health, and cardiovascular health.
- Red bell peppers, cucumbers, and red onions are low in potassium and provide vitamins, minerals, and antioxidants, promoting immune function and reducing inflammation.
- Spinach is rich in iron, calcium, and vitamin K, supporting blood and bone health.
- Avocado adds healthy fats and potassium, which may help lower blood pressure and reduce the risk of heart disease.

Preparation Time: Approximately 15 minutes.

3: Quinoa Salad with Roasted Vegetables

Ingredients:

For the salad:

- 1 cup quinoa, rinsed
- 2 cups water or low-sodium vegetable broth

- 2 cups mixed vegetables (such as bell peppers, zucchini, cherry tomatoes)
- 1 tablespoon olive oil
- Salt and pepper to taste

For the dressing:

- 2 tablespoons lemon juice
- 1 tablespoon olive oil
- 1 teaspoon Dijon mustard
- 1 clove garlic, minced
- Salt and pepper to taste

Optional toppings:

- Fresh herbs (such as parsley or basil)
- Toasted nuts or seeds (such as almonds or pumpkin seeds)
- Vegan feta cheese (optional)

Detailed Instructions:

- Preheat the oven to 400°F (200°C).
- In a saucepan, combine the quinoa and water or vegetable broth. Bring to a boil, then reduce heat to low, cover, and simmer for 15-20 minutes or until

- quinoa is cooked and liquid is absorbed. Remove from heat and let it cool slightly.
- While the quinoa is cooking, spread the mixed vegetables on a baking sheet. Drizzle with olive oil and season with salt and pepper. Roast in the preheated oven for 20-25 minutes or until vegetables are tender and slightly caramelized.
- In a small bowl, whisk together the lemon juice, olive oil, Dijon mustard, minced garlic, salt, and pepper to make the dressing.
- In a large mixing bowl, combine the cooked quinoa, roasted vegetables, and dressing. Toss until well coated.
- Divide the quinoa salad into serving bowls.
- Top with fresh herbs, toasted nuts or seeds, and vegan feta cheese if desired.
- Serve warm or at room temperature.

Health Benefits:

- Quinoa is a complete protein and a good source of fiber, supporting muscle health and digestive health.

- Mixed vegetables provide vitamins, minerals, and antioxidants, promoting immune function and reducing inflammation.
- Olive oil contains heart-healthy monounsaturated fats and antioxidants, supporting cardiovascular health and reducing oxidative stress.
- Lemon juice adds flavor and provides vitamin C, which aids in iron absorption and supports collagen production.

Preparation Time: Approximately 45 minutes.

4: Vegan Buddha Bowl

Ingredients:

For the base:

- 1 cup cooked quinoa or brown rice
- 1 cup mixed greens (such as spinach or kale)
- 1/2 cup cooked black beans
- 1/2 cup roasted sweet potatoes, diced
- 1/4 cup shredded carrots
- 1/4 cup sliced cucumber

For the tahini dressing:

- 2 tablespoons tahini
- 1 tablespoon lemon juice
- 1 tablespoon water
- 1 teaspoon maple syrup or agave syrup
- 1/2 teaspoon minced garlic
- Salt and pepper to taste

Optional toppings:

- Avocado slices
- Cherry tomatoes
- Sliced radishes
- Sprouts or microgreens

Detailed Instructions:

- Arrange the cooked quinoa or brown rice, mixed greens, cooked black beans, roasted sweet potatoes, shredded carrots, and sliced cucumber in serving bowls.
- In a small bowl, whisk together the tahini, lemon juice, water, maple syrup or agave syrup, minced

garlic, salt, and pepper to make the dressing. Adjust the consistency by adding more water if needed.
- Drizzle the tahini dressing over the Buddha bowls.
- Top with optional toppings such as avocado slices, cherry tomatoes, sliced radishes, and sprouts or microgreens.
- Serve immediately and enjoy!

Health Benefits:

- Quinoa or brown rice provides complex carbohydrates and fiber, promoting satiety and digestive health.
- Mixed greens, sweet potatoes, carrots, and cucumbers are rich in vitamins, minerals, and antioxidants, supporting immune function and reducing inflammation.
- Black beans are a good source of plant-based protein, fiber, and folate, promoting muscle health, digestive health, and cardiovascular health.
- Tahini is a source of healthy fats, protein, and calcium, supporting heart health, bone health, and muscle function.

Preparation Time: Approximately 30 minutes (if ingredients are pre-cooked).

5: Stuffed Bell Peppers with Quinoa and Black Beans

Ingredients:

- 4 large bell peppers (any color)
- 1 cup cooked quinoa
- 1 cup cooked black beans
- 1/2 cup corn kernels (fresh, frozen, or canned)
- 1/2 cup diced tomatoes
- 1/4 cup diced red onion
- 1/4 cup chopped cilantro
- 1 teaspoon ground cumin
- 1/2 teaspoon chili powder
- Salt and pepper to taste
- 1/4 cup shredded vegan cheese (optional)

Detailed Instructions:

- Preheat the oven to 375°F (190°C).
- Slice the tops off the bell peppers and remove the seeds and membranes.

- In a large mixing bowl, combine cooked quinoa, black beans, corn kernels, diced tomatoes, diced red onion, chopped cilantro, ground cumin, chili powder, salt, and pepper. Mix well.
- Stuff each bell pepper with the quinoa and black bean mixture, pressing down gently to fill.
- Place the stuffed bell peppers in a baking dish, standing upright.
- If using shredded vegan cheese, sprinkle it over the top of each stuffed bell pepper.
- Cover the baking dish with aluminum foil and bake in the preheated oven for 30-35 minutes, or until the bell peppers are tender.
- Remove from the oven and let cool slightly before serving.

Health Benefits:

- Bell peppers are low in potassium and provide vitamin C, which supports immune function and collagen production.
- Quinoa is a good source of plant-based protein and fiber, promoting muscle health and digestive health.

- Black beans are rich in protein, fiber, and folate, supporting satiety, digestive health, and cardiovascular health.
- Tomatoes are rich in antioxidants like lycopene, which may help reduce the risk of certain chronic diseases.

Preparation Time: Approximately 45 minutes.

6: Mediterranean Chickpea Salad

Ingredients:

- 2 cups cooked chickpeas (or 1 can, rinsed and drained)
- 1 cup diced cucumber
- 1 cup diced tomatoes
- 1/4 cup diced red onion
- 1/4 cup chopped fresh parsley
- 1/4 cup chopped fresh mint (optional)
- 2 tablespoons extra virgin olive oil
- 1 tablespoon lemon juice
- 1 clove garlic, minced
- Salt and pepper to taste

Detailed Instructions:

- In a large mixing bowl, combine cooked chickpeas, diced cucumber, diced tomatoes, diced red onion, chopped fresh parsley, and chopped fresh mint (if using).
- In a small bowl, whisk together extra virgin olive oil, lemon juice, minced garlic, salt, and pepper to make the dressing.
- Pour the dressing over the chickpea salad and toss until well combined.
- Let the salad marinate in the refrigerator for at least 30 minutes to allow the flavors to meld.
- Serve chilled as a side dish or main course.

Health Benefits:

- Chickpeas are a good source of plant-based protein, fiber, and folate, promoting satiety, digestive health, and cardiovascular health.
- Cucumbers are low in potassium and provide hydration and vitamin K, which supports bone health and blood clotting.

- Tomatoes are rich in antioxidants like lycopene, which may help reduce the risk of certain chronic diseases.
- Olive oil is a source of heart-healthy monounsaturated fats and antioxidants, supporting cardiovascular health and reducing inflammation.

Preparation Time: Approximately 15 minutes (plus marinating time).

7: Vegan Lentil Salad

Ingredients:

- 1 cup cooked green or brown lentils
- 1 cup diced cucumber
- 1 cup diced bell peppers (any color)
- 1/4 cup diced red onion
- 1/4 cup chopped fresh parsley
- 2 tablespoons lemon juice
- 1 tablespoon extra virgin olive oil
- 1 teaspoon Dijon mustard
- 1 clove garlic, minced
- Salt and pepper to taste

Detailed Instructions:

- In a large mixing bowl, combine cooked lentils, diced cucumber, diced bell peppers, diced red onion, and chopped fresh parsley.
- In a small bowl, whisk together lemon juice, extra virgin olive oil, Dijon mustard, minced garlic, salt, and pepper to make the dressing.
- Pour the dressing over the lentil salad and toss until well combined.
- Let the salad marinate in the refrigerator for at least 30 minutes to allow the flavors to meld.
- Serve chilled as a side dish or main course.

Health Benefits:

- Lentils are a good source of plant-based protein, fiber, and iron, promoting muscle health, digestive health, and energy levels.
- Cucumbers are low in potassium and provide hydration and vitamin K, which supports bone health and blood clotting.

- Bell peppers are rich in vitamin C and antioxidants, supporting immune function and reducing inflammation.
- Olive oil is a source of heart-healthy monounsaturated fats and antioxidants, supporting cardiovascular health and reducing inflammation.

Preparation Time: Approximately 15 minutes (plus marinating time).

8: Vegan Mediterranean Wrap

Ingredients:

- 4 whole grain wraps or tortillas
- 1 cup cooked quinoa
- 1 cup canned chickpeas, rinsed and drained
- 1/2 cup sliced cherry tomatoes
- 1/2 cup diced cucumber
- 1/4 cup diced red onion
- 1/4 cup sliced black olives
- 1/4 cup chopped fresh parsley
- 2 tablespoons lemon juice
- 2 tablespoons extra virgin olive oil
- Salt and pepper to taste

- Hummus for spreading (optional)

Detailed Instructions:

- In a large mixing bowl, combine cooked quinoa, canned chickpeas, sliced cherry tomatoes, diced cucumber, diced red onion, sliced black olives, chopped fresh parsley, lemon juice, extra virgin olive oil, salt, and pepper. Mix well.
- Warm the whole grain wraps or tortillas according to package instructions.
- Spread a layer of hummus (if using) onto each wrap or tortilla.
- Spoon the quinoa and chickpea mixture onto the wraps or tortillas.
- Roll up the wraps tightly, folding in the sides as you go.
- Slice the wraps in half diagonally and serve.

Health Benefits:

- Quinoa is a complete protein and a good source of fiber, promoting muscle health and digestive health.

- Chickpeas are rich in plant-based protein, fiber, and folate, supporting satiety, digestive health, and cardiovascular health.
- Cherry tomatoes and cucumbers are low in potassium and provide vitamins, minerals, and antioxidants, promoting immune function and reducing inflammation.
- Olives and olive oil provide healthy fats and antioxidants, supporting heart health and reducing oxidative stress.

Preparation Time: Approximately 20 minutes.

9: Vegan Mediterranean Pasta Salad

Ingredients:

- 8 ounces whole wheat pasta (penne or fusilli)
- 1 cup cherry tomatoes, halved
- 1 cup diced cucumber
- 1/2 cup sliced black olives
- 1/4 cup diced red onion
- 1/4 cup chopped fresh parsley
- 2 tablespoons lemon juice
- 2 tablespoons extra virgin olive oil

- 1 clove garlic, minced
- 1 teaspoon dried oregano
- Salt and pepper to taste
- Vegan feta cheese, crumbled (optional)

Detailed Instructions:

- Cook the whole wheat pasta according to package instructions until al dente. Drain and rinse under cold water to cool.
- In a large mixing bowl, combine the cooked pasta, cherry tomatoes, diced cucumber, sliced black olives, diced red onion, and chopped fresh parsley.
- In a small bowl, whisk together lemon juice, extra virgin olive oil, minced garlic, dried oregano, salt, and pepper to make the dressing.
- Pour the dressing over the pasta salad and toss until well combined.
- If using, sprinkle crumbled vegan feta cheese over the top of the salad.
- Serve chilled as a side dish or main course.

Health Benefits:

- Whole wheat pasta provides complex carbohydrates and fiber, promoting satiety and digestive health.
- Cherry tomatoes and cucumbers are low in potassium and provide vitamins, minerals, and antioxidants, supporting immune function and reducing inflammation.
- Black olives are a source of healthy fats and antioxidants, supporting heart health and reducing oxidative stress.
- Olive oil is a source of heart-healthy monounsaturated fats and antioxidants, supporting cardiovascular health and reducing inflammation.

Preparation Time: Approximately 20 minutes.

10: Vegan Bean and Vegetable Soup

Ingredients:

- 1 tablespoon olive oil
- 1 cup diced onion
- 1 cup diced carrot
- 1 cup diced celery

- 3 cloves garlic, minced
- 4 cups low-sodium vegetable broth
- 2 cups diced tomatoes (fresh or canned)
- 2 cups cooked beans (such as kidney beans or cannellini beans)
- 2 cups chopped kale or spinach
- 1 teaspoon dried thyme
- 1 teaspoon dried rosemary
- Salt and pepper to taste
- Fresh lemon juice (optional)

Detailed Instructions:

- Heat olive oil in a large pot over medium heat. Add diced onion, carrot, and celery. Cook until vegetables are softened, about 5-7 minutes.
- Add minced garlic and cook for an additional 1-2 minutes until fragrant.
- Pour in the vegetable broth and diced tomatoes. Bring to a simmer.
- Add cooked beans, chopped kale or spinach, dried thyme, and dried rosemary to the pot. Stir to combine.

- Simmer the soup for 15-20 minutes until the vegetables are tender.
- Season with salt and pepper to taste. Add a squeeze of fresh lemon juice if desired for brightness.
- Serve hot with whole grain bread or crackers.

Health Benefits:

- Beans are rich in plant-based protein, fiber, and minerals, promoting muscle health, digestive health, and energy levels.
- Carrots, celery, tomatoes, and kale/spinach provide vitamins, minerals, and antioxidants, supporting immune function and reducing inflammation.
- Olive oil adds healthy fats and antioxidants, supporting heart health and reducing oxidative stress.
- Fresh lemon juice provides vitamin C and adds acidity and flavor to the soup.

Preparation Time: Approximately 30 minutes.

CKD Stage 4 Dinner Recipes for Vegans

1: Vegan Chickpea Curry

Ingredients:

- 1 tablespoon olive oil
- 1 cup diced onion
- 2 cloves garlic, minced
- 1 tablespoon grated ginger
- 1 tablespoon curry powder
- 1 teaspoon ground cumin
- 1 teaspoon ground coriander
- 1/2 teaspoon turmeric powder
- 1/4 teaspoon cayenne pepper (optional, adjust to taste)
- 1 can (15 ounces) chickpeas, rinsed and drained
- 1 can (14 ounces) diced tomatoes
- 1 cup coconut milk
- Salt and pepper to taste
- Fresh cilantro for garnish (optional)

Detailed Instructions:

- Heat olive oil in a large skillet over medium heat. Add diced onion and cook until softened, about 5 minutes.
- Add minced garlic and grated ginger to the skillet. Cook for an additional 1-2 minutes until fragrant.
- Stir in curry powder, ground cumin, ground coriander, turmeric powder, and cayenne pepper (if using). Cook for 1 minute until spices are toasted and fragrant.
- Add chickpeas, diced tomatoes, and coconut milk to the skillet. Stir to combine.
- Bring the mixture to a simmer, then reduce heat to low and cover. Let it simmer for 15-20 minutes, stirring occasionally, until the sauce thickens and flavors meld.
- Season with salt and pepper to taste.
- Serve the chickpea curry hot, garnished with fresh cilantro if desired. Serve with cooked brown rice or quinoa.

Health Benefits:

- Chickpeas are rich in plant-based protein, fiber, and folate, promoting satiety, digestive health, and cardiovascular health.
- Onions, garlic, and ginger provide antioxidants and anti-inflammatory compounds, supporting immune function and reducing inflammation.
- Tomatoes are rich in vitamins, minerals, and antioxidants like lycopene, which may help reduce the risk of certain chronic diseases.
- Coconut milk adds creaminess and provides medium-chain triglycerides (MCTs), which may have potential benefits for brain health and weight management.

Preparation Time: Approximately 30 minutes.

2: Vegan Lentil Shepherd's Pie

Ingredients:

For the lentil filling:

- 1 cup green or brown lentils, rinsed
- 2 cups vegetable broth

- 1 tablespoon olive oil
- 1 cup diced onion
- 1 cup diced carrots
- 1 cup diced celery
- 2 cloves garlic, minced
- 1 teaspoon dried thyme
- 1 teaspoon dried rosemary
- Salt and pepper to taste

For the mashed potato topping:

- 2 large potatoes, peeled and diced
- 1/4 cup unsweetened almond milk
- 2 tablespoons vegan butter
- Salt and pepper to taste

Detailed Instructions:

- In a saucepan, combine the rinsed lentils and vegetable broth. Bring to a boil, then reduce heat to low and simmer for 20-25 minutes until lentils are tender and most of the liquid is absorbed.
- While the lentils are cooking, prepare the mashed potato topping. Place the diced potatoes in a pot of

water and bring to a boil. Cook for 10-15 minutes until potatoes are tender. Drain the potatoes and return them to the pot.
- Mash the potatoes using a potato masher or fork. Add almond milk, vegan butter, salt, and pepper. Continue mashing until smooth and creamy. Set aside.
- Preheat the oven to 375°F (190°C).
- In a large skillet, heat olive oil over medium heat. Add diced onion, carrots, and celery. Cook until vegetables are softened, about 5-7 minutes.
- Add minced garlic, dried thyme, dried rosemary, salt, and pepper to the skillet. Cook for an additional 1-2 minutes until fragrant.
- Stir in the cooked lentils until well combined. Transfer the lentil filling to a baking dish.
- Spread the mashed potato topping over the lentil filling, smoothing it out with a spatula.
- Bake in the preheated oven for 20-25 minutes until the top is golden brown and the filling is bubbly.
- Remove from the oven and let it cool slightly before serving.

Health Benefits:

- Lentils are rich in plant-based protein, fiber, and iron, promoting muscle health, digestive health, and energy levels.
- Potatoes are a good source of carbohydrates, vitamins, and minerals like potassium and vitamin C, supporting energy levels and immune function.
- Carrots and celery provide vitamins, minerals, and antioxidants, promoting immune function and reducing inflammation.
- Olive oil and vegan butter add healthy fats and flavor to the dish without significantly increasing sodium or phosphorus content.

Preparation Time: Approximately 60 minutes.

3: Vegan Quinoa Stuffed Bell Peppers

Ingredients:

- 4 large bell peppers (any color)
- 1 cup quinoa, rinsed
- 2 cups vegetable broth
- 1 tablespoon olive oil

- 1 cup diced onion
- 1 cup diced zucchini
- 1 cup diced tomatoes
- 1 cup cooked black beans
- 2 cloves garlic, minced
- 1 teaspoon ground cumin
- 1 teaspoon chili powder
- Salt and pepper to taste
- Fresh cilantro for garnish (optional)

Detailed Instructions:

- Preheat the oven to 375°F (190°C).
- Cut the tops off the bell peppers and remove the seeds and membranes.
- In a saucepan, bring the vegetable broth to a boil. Add quinoa, reduce heat to low, cover, and simmer for 15-20 minutes or until quinoa is cooked and liquid is absorbed.
- In a large skillet, heat olive oil over medium heat. Add diced onion and cook until softened, about 5 minutes.

- Add minced garlic, diced zucchini, diced tomatoes, cooked black beans, ground cumin, chili powder, salt, and pepper to the skillet. Cook for an additional 5-7 minutes until vegetables are tender.
- Stir in the cooked quinoa and mix until well combined.
- Stuff each bell pepper with the quinoa and vegetable mixture.
- Place the stuffed bell peppers in a baking dish. Cover with foil and bake for 25-30 minutes.
- Remove foil and bake for an additional 10-15 minutes until the peppers are tender.
- Garnish with fresh cilantro before serving.

Health Benefits:

- Bell peppers are low in potassium and rich in vitamin C and antioxidants, supporting immune function and reducing inflammation.
- Quinoa provides plant-based protein, fiber, and essential nutrients, promoting muscle health and digestive health.

- Zucchini is low in potassium and high in water content, contributing to hydration and providing vitamins and minerals.
- Black beans are a good source of plant-based protein, fiber, and folate, supporting satiety, digestive health, and cardiovascular health.

Preparation Time: Approximately 60 minutes.

4: Vegan Lentil and Vegetable Stir-Fry

Ingredients:

- 1 cup dried green lentils, rinsed
- 2 cups water
- 2 tablespoons soy sauce or tamari
- 1 tablespoon rice vinegar
- 1 tablespoon maple syrup or agave syrup
- 1 tablespoon cornstarch
- 1 tablespoon sesame oil
- 2 cloves garlic, minced
- 1 tablespoon grated ginger
- 1 cup sliced bell peppers (any color)
- 1 cup sliced carrots

- 1 cup broccoli florets
- 1 cup sliced mushrooms
- Cooked brown rice or quinoa for serving

Detailed Instructions:

- In a saucepan, combine the rinsed lentils and water. Bring to a boil, then reduce heat to low, cover, and simmer for 20-25 minutes or until lentils are tender. Drain any excess liquid.
- In a small bowl, whisk together soy sauce or tamari, rice vinegar, maple syrup or agave syrup, and cornstarch to make the sauce. Set aside.
- Heat sesame oil in a large skillet or wok over medium heat. Add minced garlic and grated ginger, and cook for 1-2 minutes until fragrant.
- Add sliced bell peppers, carrots, broccoli florets, and mushrooms to the skillet. Stir-fry for 5-7 minutes until vegetables are tender-crisp.
- Add cooked lentils to the skillet and pour the sauce over the vegetables and lentils. Stir well to coat everything evenly.

- Cook for an additional 2-3 minutes until the sauce thickens.
- Serve the lentil and vegetable stir-fry hot over cooked brown rice or quinoa.

Health Benefits:

- Lentils are a good source of plant-based protein, fiber, and iron, supporting muscle health, digestive health, and energy levels.
- Bell peppers, carrots, broccoli, and mushrooms provide vitamins, minerals, and antioxidants, supporting immune function and reducing inflammation.
- Soy sauce or tamari adds flavor and provides essential amino acids, supporting muscle repair and growth.
- Sesame oil adds flavor and healthy fats, contributing to satiety and promoting heart health.

Preparation Time: Approximately 40 minutes.

5: Vegan Eggplant and Lentil Moussaka

Ingredients:

For the lentil filling:

- 1 cup dried green lentils, rinsed
- 2 cups vegetable broth
- 1 tablespoon olive oil
- 1 cup diced onion
- 2 cloves garlic, minced
- 1 teaspoon dried oregano
- 1 teaspoon dried thyme
- 1 teaspoon ground cumin
- 1 can (14 ounces) diced tomatoes
- Salt and pepper to taste

For the eggplant layers:

- 2 large eggplants, sliced lengthwise into 1/4-inch thick slices
- Olive oil for brushing

For the topping:

- 2 cups unsweetened almond milk

- 1/4 cup cornstarch
- 1/4 cup nutritional yeast
- 1/2 teaspoon garlic powder
- Salt and pepper to taste

Detailed Instructions:

- Preheat the oven to 375°F (190°C).
- In a saucepan, combine the rinsed lentils and vegetable broth. Bring to a boil, then reduce heat to low, cover, and simmer for 20-25 minutes or until lentils are tender and most of the liquid is absorbed.
- In a skillet, heat olive oil over medium heat. Add diced onion and cook until softened, about 5 minutes. Add minced garlic, dried oregano, dried thyme, and ground cumin. Cook for an additional 1-2 minutes until fragrant.
- Stir in diced tomatoes and cooked lentils. Season with salt and pepper to taste. Simmer for 10 minutes to allow flavors to meld.
- Meanwhile, brush eggplant slices with olive oil on both sides and arrange them in a single layer on a baking sheet. Bake for 15-20 minutes until tender.

- In a saucepan, whisk together almond milk, cornstarch, nutritional yeast, garlic powder, salt, and pepper. Cook over medium heat, stirring constantly, until the mixture thickens.
- To assemble, spread half of the lentil mixture in the bottom of a baking dish. Layer half of the baked eggplant slices on top. Repeat with the remaining lentil mixture and eggplant slices.
- Pour the thickened almond milk mixture evenly over the top.
- Bake for 25-30 minutes until the topping is golden brown and bubbly.
- Let it cool for a few minutes before serving.

Health Benefits:

- Lentils are a good source of plant-based protein, fiber, and folate, promoting satiety, digestive health, and cardiovascular health.
- Eggplants are low in potassium and provide fiber and antioxidants, supporting digestive health and reducing inflammation.

- Nutritional yeast adds a cheesy flavor and provides vitamin B12, which is important for nerve function and energy metabolism.
- Almond milk is low in potassium and contains healthy fats and vitamin E, supporting heart health and skin health.

Preparation Time: Approximately 90 minutes.

6: Vegan Mediterranean Stuffed Acorn Squash

Ingredients:

- 3 acorn squash, halved and seeds removed
- 1 cup quinoa, rinsed
- 2 cups vegetable broth
- 1 tablespoon olive oil
- 1 cup diced onion
- 1 cup diced bell peppers (any color)
- 1 cup diced zucchini
- 1 cup diced tomatoes
- 1/4 cup sliced black olives
- 2 cloves garlic, minced
- 1 teaspoon dried oregano

- 1 teaspoon dried basil
- Salt and pepper to taste
- Fresh parsley for garnish (optional)

Detailed Instructions:

- Preheat the oven to 375°F (190°C).
- Place the halved acorn squash on a baking sheet, cut side up. Brush the flesh with olive oil and sprinkle with salt and pepper. Roast in the preheated oven for 30-40 minutes until tender.
- In a saucepan, combine the rinsed quinoa and vegetable broth. Bring to a boil, then reduce heat to low, cover, and simmer for 15-20 minutes or until quinoa is cooked and liquid is absorbed.
- In a skillet, heat olive oil over medium heat. Add diced onion and cook until softened, about 5 minutes. Add diced bell peppers, diced zucchini, diced tomatoes, sliced black olives, minced garlic, dried oregano, dried basil, salt, and pepper. Cook for an additional 5-7 minutes until vegetables are tender.
- Stir in cooked quinoa and mix until well combined.

- Once the acorn squash halves are tender, fill each half with the quinoa and vegetable mixture.
- Return the stuffed squash to the oven and bake for an additional 10-15 minutes to heat through.
- Garnish with fresh parsley before serving.

Health Benefits:

- Acorn squash is low in potassium and provides vitamins A, C, and B vitamins, supporting immune function, skin health, and energy metabolism.
- Quinoa is a complete protein and a good source of fiber and essential nutrients, promoting muscle health and digestive health.
- Bell peppers, zucchini, tomatoes, and olives provide vitamins, minerals, and antioxidants, supporting immune function and reducing inflammation.
- Olive oil adds healthy fats and flavor to the dish without significantly increasing sodium or phosphorus content.

Preparation Time: Approximately 60 minutes.

7: Vegan Lentil Shepherd's Pie

Ingredients:

For the lentil filling:

- 1 cup dried green lentils, rinsed
- 2 cups vegetable broth
- 1 tablespoon olive oil
- 1 cup diced onion
- 1 cup diced carrots
- 1 cup diced celery
- 2 cloves garlic, minced
- 1 teaspoon dried thyme
- 1 teaspoon dried rosemary
- 1 can (14 ounces) diced tomatoes
- Salt and pepper to taste

For the mashed potato topping:

- 4 large potatoes, peeled and diced
- 1/4 cup unsweetened almond milk
- 2 tablespoons vegan butter
- Salt and pepper to taste

Detailed Instructions:

- Preheat the oven to 375°F (190°C).
- In a saucepan, combine the rinsed lentils and vegetable broth. Bring to a boil, then reduce heat to low, cover, and simmer for 20-25 minutes or until lentils are tender and most of the liquid is absorbed.
- Meanwhile, in a separate pot, cook the diced potatoes in boiling water until tender, about 10-15 minutes.
- In a skillet, heat olive oil over medium heat. Add diced onion, carrots, and celery. Cook until vegetables are softened, about 5-7 minutes. Add minced garlic, dried thyme, and dried rosemary. Cook for an additional 1-2 minutes until fragrant.
- Stir in diced tomatoes and cooked lentils. Season with salt and pepper to taste. Simmer for 10 minutes to allow flavors to meld.
- Drain the cooked potatoes and return them to the pot. Mash the potatoes with almond milk, vegan butter, salt, and pepper until smooth and creamy.
- Transfer the lentil filling to a baking dish. Spread the mashed potatoes evenly over the top.

- Bake in the preheated oven for 25-30 minutes until the mashed potato topping is golden brown and the filling is bubbly.
- Let it cool for a few minutes before serving.

Health Benefits:

- Lentils are a good source of plant-based protein, fiber, and folate, promoting satiety, digestive health, and cardiovascular health.
- Potatoes are a good source of carbohydrates, vitamins, and minerals like potassium and vitamin C, supporting energy levels and immune function.
- Carrots and celery provide vitamins, minerals, and antioxidants, promoting immune function and reducing inflammation.
- Almond milk adds creaminess and provides calcium, supporting bone health and muscle function.

Preparation Time: Approximately 60 minutes.

8: Vegan Mediterranean Stuffed Portobello Mushrooms

Ingredients:

- 4 large portobello mushrooms, stems removed and gills scraped out
- 1 cup cooked quinoa
- 1 cup diced tomatoes
- 1/2 cup diced red onion
- 1/2 cup diced bell peppers (any color)
- 1/4 cup sliced black olives
- 2 cloves garlic, minced
- 2 tablespoons chopped fresh parsley
- 2 tablespoons olive oil
- 1 tablespoon balsamic vinegar
- Salt and pepper to taste

Detailed Instructions:

- Preheat the oven to 375°F (190°C).
- In a mixing bowl, combine cooked quinoa, diced tomatoes, diced red onion, diced bell peppers, sliced black olives, minced garlic, chopped parsley, olive

oil, and balsamic vinegar. Season with salt and pepper to taste.

- Place the portobello mushrooms on a baking sheet, gill side up.
- Divide the quinoa mixture evenly among the portobello mushrooms, pressing it down gently.
- Bake in the preheated oven for 20-25 minutes until the mushrooms are tender and the filling is heated through.
- Remove from the oven and let it cool for a few minutes before serving.

Health Benefits:

- Portobello mushrooms are low in calories and carbohydrates and provide protein, fiber, and essential nutrients like B vitamins and selenium, supporting immune function and energy metabolism.
- Quinoa is a complete protein and a good source of fiber and essential nutrients, promoting muscle health and digestive health.
- Tomatoes, red onions, bell peppers, olives, and parsley provide vitamins, minerals, and antioxidants,

supporting immune function and reducing inflammation.
- Olive oil adds healthy fats and flavor to the dish without significantly increasing sodium or phosphorus content.

Preparation Time: Approximately 30 minutes.

9: Vegan Lentil and Vegetable Soup

Ingredients:

- 1 tablespoon olive oil
- 1 cup diced onion
- 1 cup diced carrots
- 1 cup diced celery
- 2 cloves garlic, minced
- 1 cup dried green lentils, rinsed
- 6 cups low-sodium vegetable broth
- 1 can (14 ounces) diced tomatoes
- 2 cups chopped spinach or kale
- 1 teaspoon dried thyme
- 1 teaspoon dried rosemary
- Salt and pepper to taste

Detailed Instructions:

- In a large pot, heat olive oil over medium heat. Add diced onion, carrots, and celery. Cook until softened, about 5-7 minutes.
- Add minced garlic and cook for an additional 1-2 minutes until fragrant.
- Stir in dried green lentils, vegetable broth, diced tomatoes (with juices), dried thyme, and dried rosemary. Bring to a boil.
- Reduce heat to low, cover, and simmer for 25-30 minutes, stirring occasionally, until lentils are tender.
- Add chopped spinach or kale to the soup during the last 5 minutes of cooking.
- Season with salt and pepper to taste.
- Serve hot with whole grain bread or crackers.

Health Benefits:

- Lentils are a good source of plant-based protein, fiber, and folate, promoting satiety, digestive health, and cardiovascular health.

- Carrots, celery, and tomatoes provide vitamins, minerals, and antioxidants, supporting immune function and reducing inflammation.
- Spinach or kale are rich in vitamins A, C, and K, as well as iron and calcium, supporting bone health, immune function, and blood clotting.
- Olive oil adds healthy fats and flavor to the soup without significantly increasing sodium or phosphorus content.

Preparation Time: Approximately 45 minutes.

10: Vegan Quinoa and Vegetable Stir-Fry

Ingredients:

- 1 cup quinoa, rinsed
- 2 cups low-sodium vegetable broth
- 2 tablespoons soy sauce or tamari
- 1 tablespoon rice vinegar
- 1 tablespoon maple syrup or agave syrup
- 1 tablespoon cornstarch
- 1 tablespoon sesame oil
- 2 cloves garlic, minced
- 1 tablespoon grated ginger

- 2 cups mixed vegetables (such as bell peppers, broccoli, carrots, snap peas)
- Salt and pepper to taste
- Chopped green onions for garnish (optional)

Detailed Instructions:

- In a saucepan, combine the rinsed quinoa and vegetable broth. Bring to a boil, then reduce heat to low, cover, and simmer for 15-20 minutes or until quinoa is cooked and liquid is absorbed.
- In a small bowl, whisk together soy sauce or tamari, rice vinegar, maple syrup or agave syrup, and cornstarch to make the sauce. Set aside.
- Heat sesame oil in a large skillet or wok over medium heat. Add minced garlic and grated ginger, and cook for 1-2 minutes until fragrant.
- Add mixed vegetables to the skillet and stir-fry for 5-7 minutes until tender-crisp.
- Stir in cooked quinoa and the sauce mixture. Cook for an additional 2-3 minutes until the sauce thickens and coats the vegetables and quinoa evenly.
- Season with salt and pepper to taste.

- Serve hot, garnished with chopped green onions if desired.

Health Benefits:

- Quinoa provides complete protein and fiber, promoting muscle health and digestive health.
- Mixed vegetables offer a variety of vitamins, minerals, and antioxidants, supporting immune function and reducing inflammation.
- Soy sauce or tamari adds flavor and provides essential amino acids, supporting muscle repair and growth.
- Sesame oil adds healthy fats and enhances the flavor of the stir-fry.

Preparation Time: Approximately 30 minutes.

CKD Stage 4 Snacks Recipes for Vegans

1: Vegan Hummus and Vegetable Platter

Ingredients:

- 1 cup cooked chickpeas (or 1 can, drained and rinsed)
- 2 tablespoons tahini
- 2 tablespoons lemon juice

- 1 clove garlic, minced
- 2 tablespoons extra virgin olive oil
- Salt and pepper to taste
- Assorted vegetables for dipping (such as carrot sticks, cucumber slices, bell pepper strips, cherry tomatoes)

Detailed Instructions:

- In a food processor, combine cooked chickpeas, tahini, lemon juice, minced garlic, extra virgin olive oil, salt, and pepper.
- Blend until smooth and creamy, adding a splash of water if needed to achieve the desired consistency.
- Transfer the hummus to a serving bowl and garnish with a drizzle of olive oil and a sprinkle of paprika or chopped fresh parsley (optional).
- Arrange assorted vegetables around the hummus in a platter or serving tray.
- Serve immediately and enjoy!

Health Benefits:

- Chickpeas are a good source of plant-based protein and fiber, promoting satiety and digestive health.
- Tahini provides healthy fats and minerals like calcium and magnesium, supporting bone health and energy metabolism.
- Assorted vegetables offer vitamins, minerals, and antioxidants, supporting immune function and reducing inflammation.
- Olive oil adds healthy monounsaturated fats and antioxidants, supporting heart health and reducing oxidative stress.

Preparation Time: Approximately 10 minutes.

2: Vegan Avocado Toast

Ingredients:

- 2 slices whole grain bread (choose low-sodium options if available)
- 1 ripe avocado
- 1 small tomato, sliced
- Fresh lemon juice

- Red pepper flakes (optional)
- Salt and pepper to taste

Detailed Instructions:

- Toast the whole grain bread slices until golden brown and crispy.
- While the bread is toasting, cut the avocado in half, remove the pit, and scoop the flesh into a small bowl.
- Mash the avocado with a fork until smooth, adding a squeeze of fresh lemon juice to prevent browning.
- Season the mashed avocado with salt and pepper to taste.
- Once the toast is ready, spread the mashed avocado evenly onto each slice.
- Top the avocado toast with sliced tomatoes and a sprinkle of red pepper flakes (if desired).
- Serve immediately and enjoy!

Health Benefits:

- Whole grain bread provides complex carbohydrates and fiber, promoting satiety and digestive health.

- Avocado is rich in healthy monounsaturated fats, vitamins, and minerals like potassium and vitamin K, supporting heart health and bone health.
- Tomatoes offer vitamins, minerals, and antioxidants like lycopene, supporting immune function and reducing inflammation.
- Lemon juice adds vitamin C and acidity to enhance flavor.

Preparation Time: Approximately 10 minutes.

3: Vegan Berry Smoothie Bowl

Ingredients:

- 1 ripe banana, frozen
- 1 cup mixed berries (such as strawberries, blueberries, raspberries)
- 1/2 cup unsweetened almond milk
- 1 tablespoon chia seeds
- 1 tablespoon almond butter (optional)
- Toppings: sliced fresh fruit, granola, shredded coconut, nuts, seeds

Detailed Instructions:

- In a blender, combine the frozen banana, mixed berries, unsweetened almond milk, chia seeds, and almond butter (if using).
- Blend until smooth and creamy, adding more almond milk if needed to reach the desired consistency.
- Pour the smoothie into a bowl.
- Top the smoothie with sliced fresh fruit, granola, shredded coconut, nuts, and seeds of your choice.
- Serve immediately with a spoon and enjoy!

Health Benefits:

- Berries are rich in vitamins, minerals, and antioxidants, supporting immune function and reducing inflammation.
- Banana adds natural sweetness and potassium, supporting heart health and muscle function.
- Chia seeds provide omega-3 fatty acids, fiber, and protein, promoting satiety, digestive health, and cardiovascular health.

- Almond milk is low in potassium and provides calcium and vitamin D, supporting bone health and muscle function.

Preparation Time: Approximately 5 minutes.

4: Vegan Antipasto Skewers

Ingredients:

- Cherry tomatoes
- Artichoke hearts, drained
- Pitted olives (such as Kalamata or green)
- Vegan mozzarella cheese, cubed
- Basil leaves
- Balsamic glaze (optional)
- Skewers or toothpicks

Detailed Instructions:

- Assemble the antipasto skewers by threading cherry tomatoes, artichoke hearts, pitted olives, vegan mozzarella cheese cubes, and basil leaves onto skewers or toothpicks in any desired order.
- Repeat until all ingredients are used and the skewers are filled.

- Arrange the skewers on a serving platter.
- Drizzle with balsamic glaze (if using) for extra flavor.
- Serve immediately or refrigerate until ready to serve.

Health Benefits:

- Cherry tomatoes are low in potassium and provide vitamins, minerals, and antioxidants, supporting immune function and reducing inflammation.
- Artichoke hearts are a good source of fiber, vitamins, and minerals like potassium and magnesium, supporting digestive health and heart health.
- Olives are rich in healthy fats and antioxidants, supporting heart health and reducing oxidative stress.
- Vegan mozzarella cheese provides protein and calcium, supporting muscle health and bone health.

Preparation Time: Approximately 15 minutes.

5: Vegan Chickpea Salad

Ingredients:

- 1 can (15 ounces) chickpeas, drained and rinsed
- 1/2 cup diced cucumber

- 1/2 cup diced bell pepper (any color)
- 1/4 cup diced red onion
- 2 tablespoons chopped fresh parsley
- 1 tablespoon extra virgin olive oil
- 1 tablespoon lemon juice
- 1 teaspoon Dijon mustard
- Salt and pepper to taste

Detailed Instructions:

- In a mixing bowl, combine the drained and rinsed chickpeas, diced cucumber, diced bell pepper, diced red onion, and chopped fresh parsley.
- In a small bowl, whisk together the extra virgin olive oil, lemon juice, Dijon mustard, salt, and pepper to make the dressing.
- Pour the dressing over the chickpea mixture and toss until well combined.
- Taste and adjust seasoning if necessary.
- Serve immediately or refrigerate until ready to serve.

Health Benefits:

- Chickpeas are a good source of plant-based protein, fiber, and folate, promoting satiety, digestive health, and cardiovascular health.
- Cucumbers are low in potassium and provide hydration and vitamins like vitamin K and vitamin C, supporting bone health and immune function.
- Bell peppers offer vitamins, minerals, and antioxidants, supporting immune function and reducing inflammation.
- Olive oil provides healthy monounsaturated fats and antioxidants, supporting heart health and reducing oxidative stress.

Preparation Time: Approximately 10 minutes.

6: Vegan Rice Cake with Almond Butter and Banana

Ingredients:

- 1 rice cake (choose low-sodium options if available)
- 1 tablespoon almond butter (or any nut or seed butter)

- 1/2 ripe banana, sliced
- Drizzle of honey or maple syrup (optional)

Detailed Instructions:

- Spread almond butter evenly over the rice cake.
- Arrange sliced banana on top of the almond butter.
- Drizzle with honey or maple syrup if desired for extra sweetness.
- Serve immediately and enjoy!

Health Benefits:

- Rice cakes provide a low-sodium and gluten-free base for the snack, offering carbohydrates for energy.
- Almond butter adds healthy fats, protein, and fiber, promoting satiety and providing essential nutrients like vitamin E and magnesium.
- Bananas are rich in potassium, vitamins, and fiber, supporting heart health, muscle function, and digestive health.
- Honey or maple syrup (if used) add natural sweetness without significantly increasing sodium or phosphorus content.

Preparation Time: Approximately 5 minutes.

7: Vegan Stuffed Mini Bell Peppers

Ingredients:

- 12 mini bell peppers
- 1 cup cooked quinoa
- 1/2 cup black beans, drained and rinsed
- 1/4 cup diced tomatoes
- 1/4 cup diced red onion
- 1/4 cup chopped fresh cilantro
- 1 tablespoon lime juice
- 1 teaspoon ground cumin
- Salt and pepper to taste
- Guacamole or salsa for dipping (optional)

Detailed Instructions:

- Preheat the oven to 375°F (190°C).
- Cut the tops off the mini bell peppers and remove the seeds and membranes.
- In a mixing bowl, combine cooked quinoa, black beans, diced tomatoes, diced red onion, chopped

fresh cilantro, lime juice, ground cumin, salt, and pepper.
- Stuff each mini bell pepper with the quinoa mixture, pressing down gently to fill.
- Place the stuffed mini bell peppers on a baking sheet lined with parchment paper.
- Bake in the preheated oven for 15-20 minutes until the peppers are tender.
- Remove from the oven and let cool slightly before serving.
- Serve with guacamole or salsa for dipping, if desired.

Health Benefits:

- Mini bell peppers are low in potassium and provide vitamins A and C, promoting immune function and reducing inflammation.
- Quinoa is a complete protein and a good source of fiber and essential nutrients, promoting muscle health and digestive health.
- Black beans provide plant-based protein, fiber, and folate, supporting satiety, digestive health, and cardiovascular health.

- Tomatoes, red onion, cilantro, and lime juice add flavor and provide vitamins, minerals, and antioxidants.

Preparation Time: Approximately 30 minutes.

8: Vegan Greek Yogurt Parfait

Ingredients:

- 1 cup unsweetened dairy-free yogurt (such as almond or coconut yogurt)
- 1/2 cup mixed berries (such as strawberries, blueberries, raspberries)
- 1/4 cup granola (choose low-sodium options if available)
- 1 tablespoon chopped nuts or seeds (such as almonds, walnuts, chia seeds)
- Drizzle of honey or maple syrup (optional)

Detailed Instructions:

- In a serving glass or bowl, layer unsweetened dairy-free yogurt, mixed berries, and granola.
- Repeat the layers until the glass or bowl is filled.
- Top with chopped nuts or seeds.

- Drizzle with honey or maple syrup if desired for extra sweetness.
- Serve immediately and enjoy!

Health Benefits:

- Dairy-free yogurt provides probiotics and is low in potassium, supporting digestive health and immune function.
- Mixed berries offer vitamins, minerals, and antioxidants, supporting immune function and reducing inflammation.
- Granola adds crunch and provides carbohydrates, fiber, and healthy fats for energy and satiety.
- Nuts or seeds offer protein, healthy fats, and essential nutrients like omega-3 fatty acids and vitamin E.

Preparation Time: Approximately 5 minutes.

9: Vegan Edamame Salad

Ingredients:

- 1 cup shelled edamame, cooked
- 1/2 cup diced cucumber
- 1/2 cup diced red bell pepper

- 2 tablespoons chopped fresh cilantro
- 1 tablespoon rice vinegar
- 1 tablespoon low-sodium soy sauce or tamari
- 1 teaspoon sesame oil
- 1 teaspoon grated ginger
- Sesame seeds for garnish (optional)

Detailed Instructions:

- In a mixing bowl, combine cooked edamame, diced cucumber, diced red bell pepper, and chopped fresh cilantro.
- In a small bowl, whisk together rice vinegar, low-sodium soy sauce or tamari, sesame oil, and grated ginger to make the dressing.
- Pour the dressing over the edamame mixture and toss until well combined.
- Garnish with sesame seeds if desired.
- Serve immediately or refrigerate until ready to serve.

Health Benefits:

- Edamame is a good source of plant-based protein, fiber, and essential nutrients like folate and iron, promoting muscle health and energy metabolism.
- Cucumber and red bell pepper provide hydration, vitamins, minerals, and antioxidants, supporting immune function and reducing inflammation.
- Fresh cilantro adds flavor and provides vitamins, minerals, and antioxidants.
- Rice vinegar, soy sauce or tamari, sesame oil, and ginger add savory and tangy flavors while providing additional health benefits.

Preparation Time: Approximately 10 minutes.

10: Vegan Chia Pudding

Ingredients:

- 1/4 cup chia seeds
- 1 cup unsweetened almond milk
- 1 tablespoon maple syrup or agave syrup
- 1/2 teaspoon vanilla extract

- Fresh fruit for topping (such as sliced strawberries, banana, kiwi)
- Chopped nuts or seeds for topping (such as almonds, walnuts, pumpkin seeds)

Detailed Instructions:

- In a mixing bowl or jar, combine chia seeds, unsweetened almond milk, maple syrup or agave syrup, and vanilla extract.
- Stir well to combine.
- Cover the bowl or jar and refrigerate for at least 2 hours or overnight, until the mixture thickens and forms a pudding-like consistency.
- Once the chia pudding is set, give it a stir.
- Serve the chia pudding in individual bowls or glasses.
- Top with fresh fruit and chopped nuts or seeds of your choice.
- Serve immediately and enjoy!

Health Benefits:

- Chia seeds are rich in omega-3 fatty acids, fiber, and protein, promoting satiety, digestive health, and cardiovascular health.
- Unsweetened almond milk is low in potassium and provides calcium and vitamin D, supporting bone health and muscle function.
- Maple syrup or agave syrup adds sweetness without significantly increasing sodium or phosphorus content.
- Fresh fruit and nuts or seeds provide vitamins, minerals, and antioxidants, adding flavor and texture to the chia pudding.

Preparation Time: Approximately 5 minutes (plus chilling time).

CONCLUSION

The CKD Stage 4 Cookbook for Vegans offers a comprehensive guide to navigating the dietary challenges of chronic kidney disease (CKD) while following a vegan lifestyle.

With its carefully crafted recipes tailored to the specific nutritional needs of individuals in Stage 4 CKD, this cookbook provides a wealth of delicious and nourishing options to support kidney health.

By emphasizing plant-based ingredients rich in essential nutrients, fiber, and antioxidants, this cookbook empowers individuals with CKD Stage 4 to make informed dietary choices that promote overall well-being.

From hearty breakfasts to satisfying dinners and everything in between, each recipe is thoughtfully designed to prioritize kidney health without compromising on flavor or variety.

The detailed instructions, ingredient lists, and health benefits provided with each recipe make it easy for individuals and their caregivers to plan and prepare meals with confidence. Whether you're seeking to manage your CKD symptoms, optimize your nutritional intake, or simply enjoy delicious vegan fare, this cookbook serves as a valuable resource on your journey toward better health.

In embracing the principles of mindful eating and nourishing your body with wholesome, plant-based foods, the CKD Stage 4 Cookbook for Vegans not only supports kidney health but also promotes a sustainable and compassionate approach to eating.

With its emphasis on creativity, flavor, and nourishment, this cookbook invites you to explore a world of delicious possibilities while taking proactive steps toward managing CKD Stage 4 with confidence and vitality.

www.ingramcontent.com/pod-product-compliance
Lightning Source LLC
Chambersburg PA
CBHW050323230526
45471CB00005B/2320